An exciting adventure that illustrates the importance of nutrition to children.

Stargold the Food Fairy

written by
Claudia Lemay, RD
illustrations by
Chris Hamilton

"Good foods build the brain;
good books expand it."

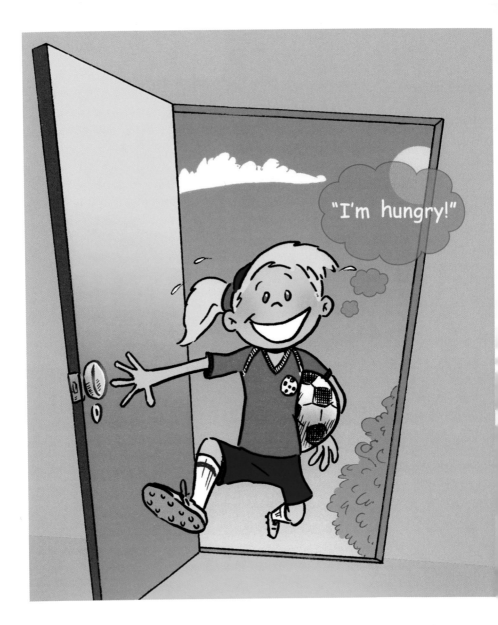

The other day, when Lucie came home from soccer practice, she was super-duper extra hungry. She ran through the kitchen door and rushed to the pantry, looking for candy.

"Oh hello, Lucie," said her mother. "I was just putting dinner on the table. It's a nice omelette full of vegetables!"

Lucie looked at the food on her plate.

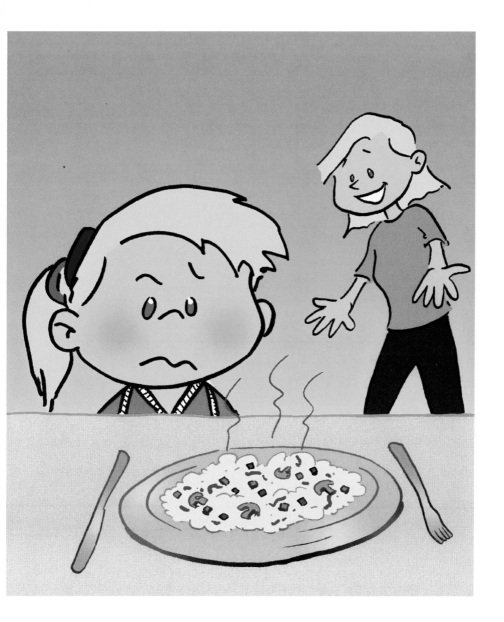

"I don't want that," she said. "I want marshmallow stew with cotton candy instead!"

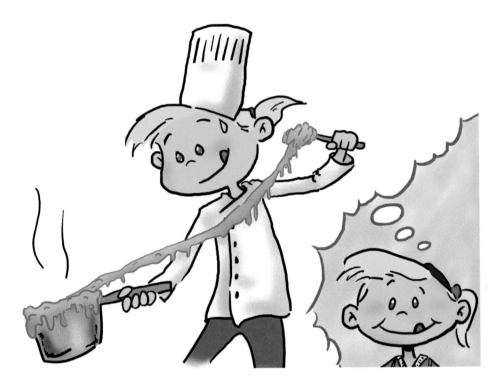

Her mother laughed. "Absolutely not, sweetie. As the parent, I choose what we eat. Now go wash your hands, please."

"That's not fair," said Lucie, scrubbing her hands at the sink. "Why don't I get to make any choices?"

"Your choices are whether you eat or not and how much you eat."

"I want to eat candy," yelled Lucie.

"But that's not what I made, sweetie," insisted her mother.

"Okay, I am going to eat in my room then," said Lucie, secretly planning to throw it out the window to the neighbour's dog, who didn't seem fussy at all.

"How am I supposed to hear about your day then? We eat together as a family every day," said her mother in her 'Mom Voice'.

Lucie got angry. She got so angry, that she ran to her room, slammed the door, and sat on her bed, sulking. She was hungry, but she did not want to eat that gross omelette! Her belly rumbled, and that's when she heard a soft 'swoosh'...

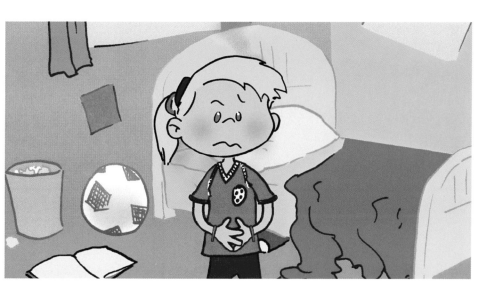

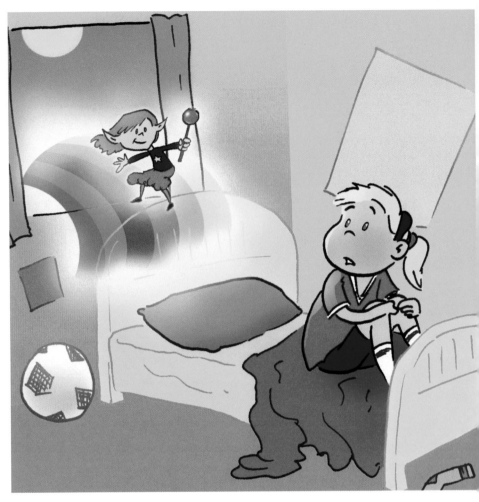

Through the window, a small creature with pointy ears had flown in, riding on a sparkling rainbow.

"Hello, Lucie," said the pointy-eared creature.

"Uh, hello," said Lucie. "Who are you?"

"My name is Stargold and I am the Food Fairy."

"What! A Food Fairy?" asked Lucie.

"I may not be as popular as my cousin, the Tooth Fairy, but my job is just as important. I help children all over the world grow strong and healthy! I want to show you Growland. Do you want to come?"

"Sure, but where did you say we are going?" asked Lucie, still hoping she might get candy.

"Growland! It's a magical place!"

"Magical? Cool! Let's go!"

Stargold took Lucie's hand and they flew out the window.

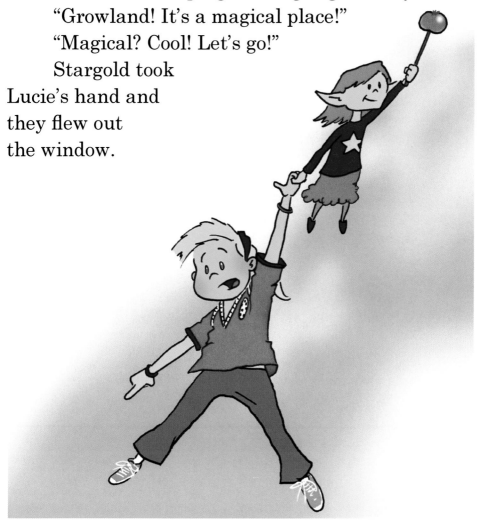

They flew over oceans and deserts, waterfalls and jungles. They soared over a giant forest and finally arrived in Growland. Lucie could see thousands of rivers, thousands of red boats, and thousands of brightly coloured houses everywhere.

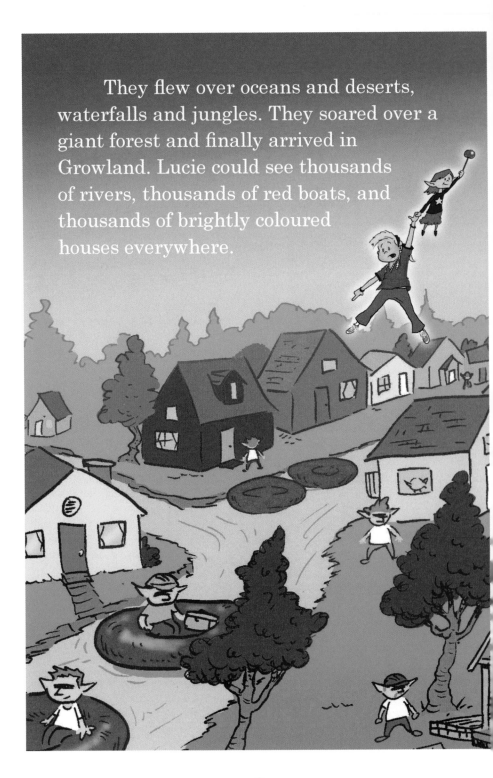

Lucie stared in amazement.

Stargold said, "Here in Growland, there are only rivers. That means we will travel around by boat."

When they landed, Stargold led Lucie to a boat and said: "Hop on! Lets go explore Growland." They both jumped in and set off down the river.

"The Elves here build magical houses," said Stargold.

"How are they magical?" Lucie asked.

"The houses here are not real. Each one is actually the body of a person in the world you live in."

"Huh? How does that work?" asked Lucie, puzzled.

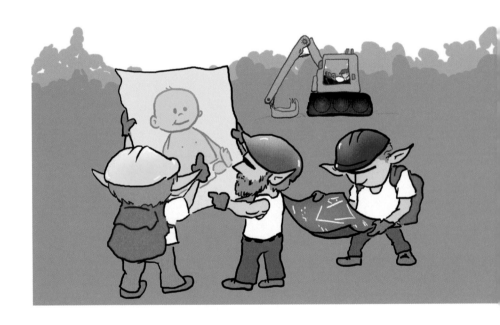

"When a mother gives birth to a baby, the Elves receive the information from the parents 'DNA' on how the baby's body is supposed to grow."

"The Elves then build the baby's body here in Growland as a house," Stargold went on, "And in your world, it grows as the baby's body."

"Wow! really?" said Lucie.

"Close your eyes, and take my hand. I have a surprise for you!"

"Oh, I love surprises," exclaimed Lucie.

Stargold brought Lucie further down the river.

"Open your eyes," she said, pointing to a cute little house. "That is YOUR house!"

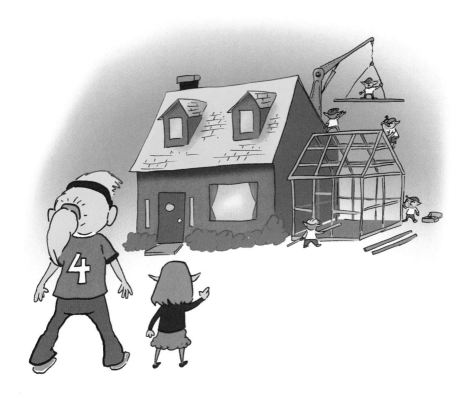

"Whoa! It looks just like me," Lucie said.

"Yes, and look how hard they are working on this one," said Stargold.

"How do the Elves build houses? " asked Lucie.

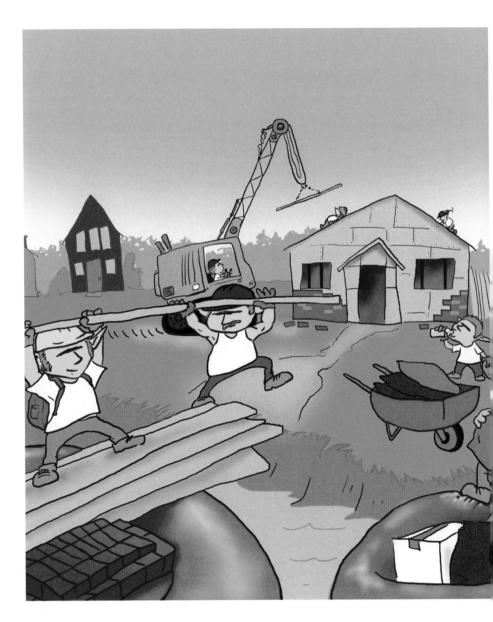

"All the necessary materials are brought in by boats to the construction site. The materials only come to the builders when that person eats something," explained Stargold.

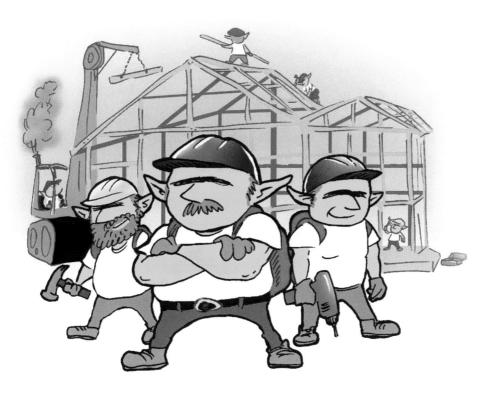

"Look! The Body Builder Elves are building the frame of an extension on your house. In your body, that would be the skeleton."

"Without the skeleton," Stargold went on, "your body would be a big blob on the ground. Now, watch this!" said Stargold, flicking her wand.

A tray magically appeared. It was full of different kinds of calcium-rich foods.

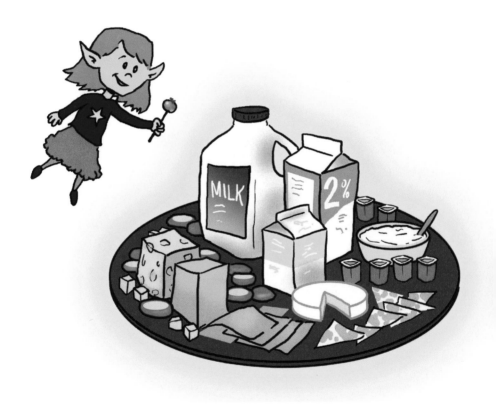

Stargold continued: "Calcium is the material needed to build your bones, just like wood is needed to build the frame of a house. Now drink some milk and watch what happens!"

Lucie took a giant gulp, and suddenly a boat came around the corner carrying large, strong boards of wood.

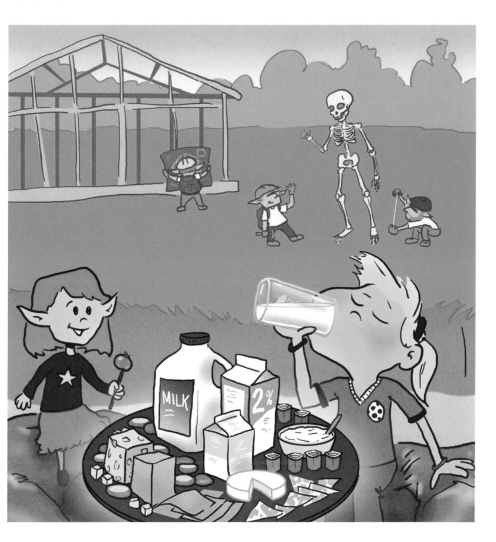

"Well done!" said Stargold. "Now the Body Builder Elves have what they need."

"Wow!" said Lucie.

"Let's see what happens next," said Stargold. She pointed to Lucie's house. "In order to make the bricks for the walls of your house, the Elves need you to eat foods that are high in protein."

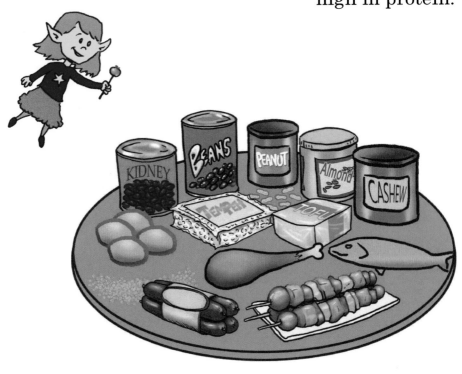

Stargold waved her wand and another tray showed up. This one was full of protein-rich foods.

"Protein is the building block of almost everything in your body – your muscles, hair, skin and even your heart."

Lucie grabbed some hard-boiled eggs and stuffed her cheeks.

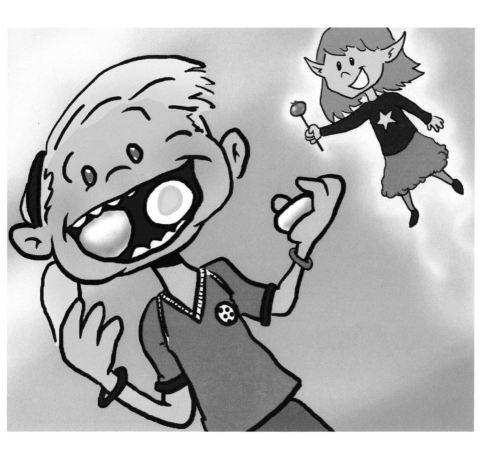

Everyone laughed. "Keep going like this, and I will have to call my aunt, the Good Manners Fairy, and start a whole other book about you, Lucie!" said Stargold, chuckling.

As Lucie chewed, a boat showed up at the dock in front of Lucie's house and the elves started unloading bricks.

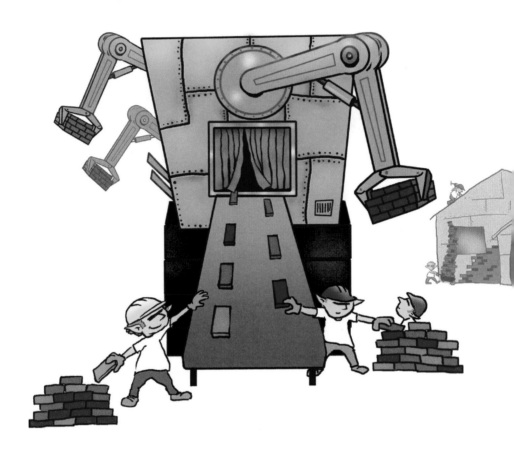

"See what just happened? Now they can build the walls of your house. With these bricks the walls will be strong, just like your muscles and your heart."

Lucie nodded, her mouth still too full of eggs to talk.

Stargold continued, "Now in order for all the parts of your body to function well together, you need your brain. The part of a house that is like your brain is the computer. You need to eat foods that are high in healthy fats so that the Geek Elves can build the computer for your house. These foods contain essential fatty acids which are the building blocks of your brain."

Stargold waved her wand and a tray with food containing healthy fats and oils appeared.

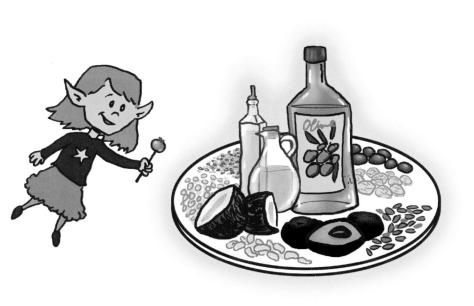

Lucie grabbed a handful of walnuts and started eating them. Stargold guided her closer to her house so she could see better.

Just then, a boat pulled up carrying computer parts that other Elves carried into Lucie's house.

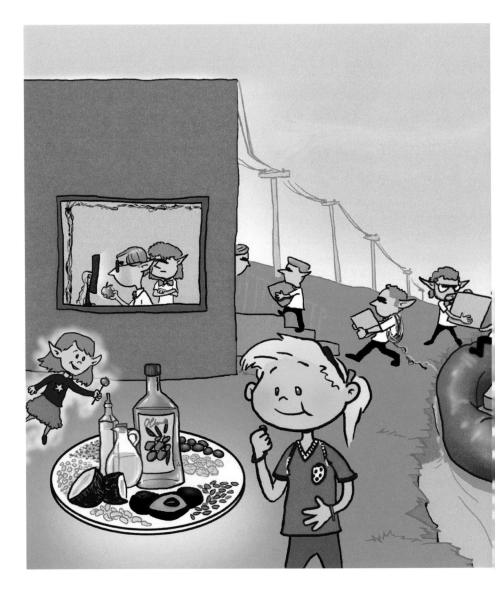

"Eating good oils ensures your brain will work well. After all, building your brain is just as important as protecting it, like you do when you wear a helmet when you go biking."

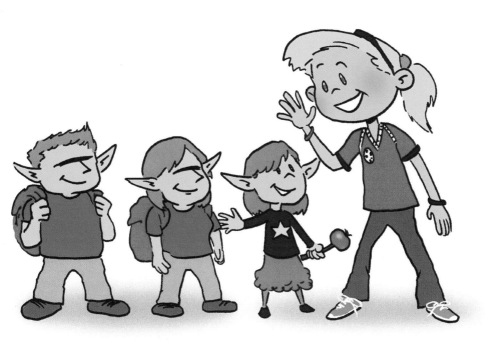

Lucie noticed two Elves walking towards them. Stargold waved them over.

"Hello! My name is Ana!" said the girl Elf.

"Hello! My name is Bolly!" said the boy Elf. "We are Junior Body Builder Elves."

"Hi, I am Lucie!" she answered.

"Could you please show Lucie what you carry in your backpacks?" asked Stargold.

"Of course," said Bolly, opening his bag for Lucie. "We carry the same things you carry in your backpack, but instead of school supplies, we bring tools."

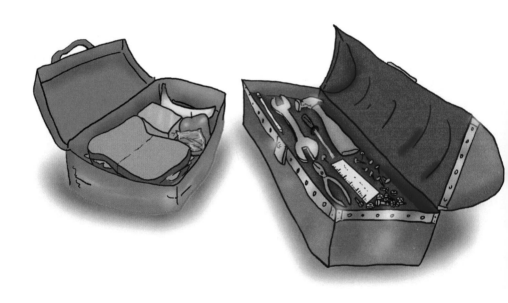

Ana continued: "When you eat whole grains, the boats bring lunch boxes for us to have the energy to build your house. Whole grains contain a lot of carbohydrates as well as vitamins and minerals. Carbohydrates give us energy, while vitamins and minerals give us tools."

"Let me show you," said Stargold.

She waved her wand and a tray with whole grain foods appeared.

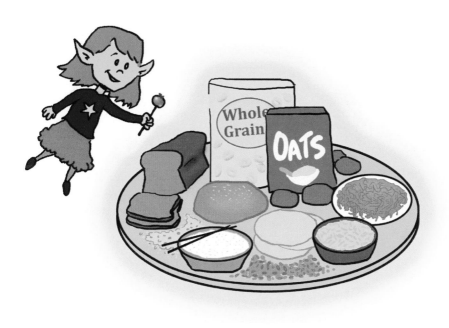

Lucie grabbed a delicious-looking whole grain roll and took a huge bite.

Right then, a boat zoomed up to the dock, and Ana and Bolly ran to fill their backpacks.

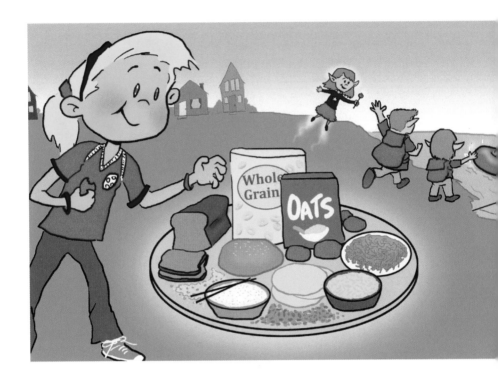

"There are other foods that contain a lot of carbohydrates: Candy, for example," said Ana, smiling.

"Yay! Stargold, make a tray of candy appear!" said Lucie.

Stargold laughed. "When you eat or drink candy, which you do when you drink soda pop, we only get lunchboxes, but zero tools! Candy doesn't have vitamins and minerals, while whole grains do. We need tools just as much as we need energy!"

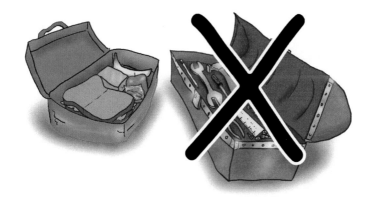

"Really?" Lucie said. "I had no idea!"

"That's why I brought you here," said Stargold. "Most kids don't know this."

"I understand now," Lucie said.

"Great. Let's go see some more."

They waved goodbye to Ana and Bolly and walked back to the river.

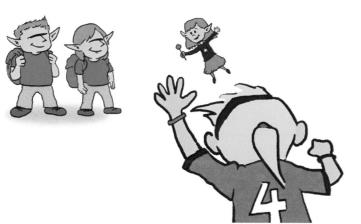

Suddenly, they heard a loud screeching noise.
Lucie looked up and saw mischievous-looking monkeys coming their way. The monkeys had climbed up onto the roof tops and started pulling shingles loose to toss at each other.

"HeeeeHeeeeHeeee!" they said snickering.

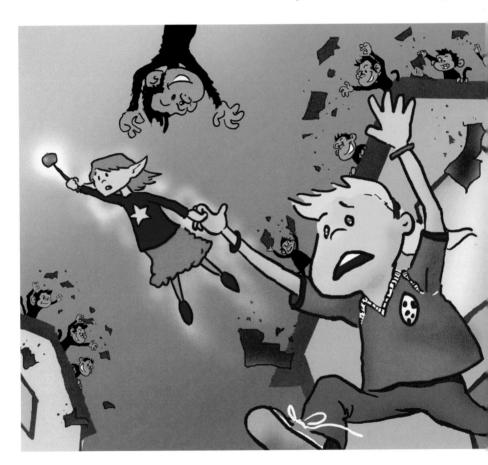

"Follow me! Quick!" Stargold yelled. "The Mayhem Monkeys are here! Let's go warn the captain!"

She grabbed Lucie's hand and they flew to the Rescue Station.

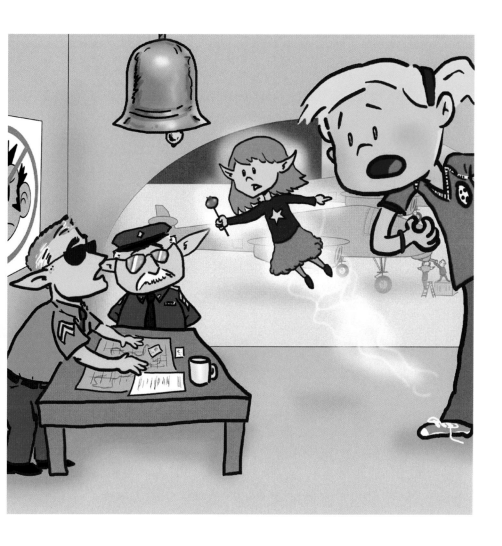

Stargold warned the Elf captain and he rang a big blue bell to alert the Pilot Elves to get to their planes. As Lucie and Stargold watched, the planes rolled out onto the runway and took off one by one.

"When the Mayhem Monkeys come, they cause so much damage to our houses!" said Stargold.

"How can we stop them?" Lucie asked.

"Lucie, this is where we need YOU! We need lasers to scare away the Mayhem Monkeys, but we only get them when you eat antioxidants from fruit and vegetables."

"Vegetables?! Ewww!" Lucie shuddered. "Vegetables are sooo gross. But if they can turn into lasers, that's pretty cool."

Stargold waved her wand and a tray full of fabulously-coloured fruit and vegetables appeared.

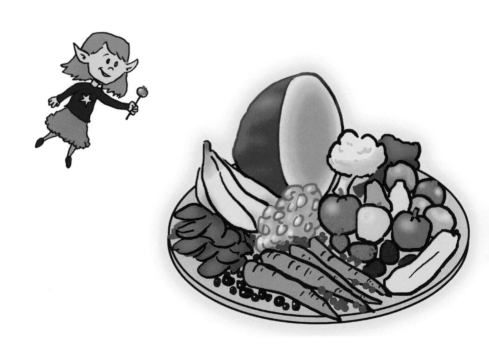

"Now come with me, I will show you!" said Stargold.

They hurried to the runway. Stargold continued: "These boxes are full of lasers. As soon as they arrive, they are loaded onto the planes. Once loaded, the pilots will be equipped to zap the mayhem monkeys."

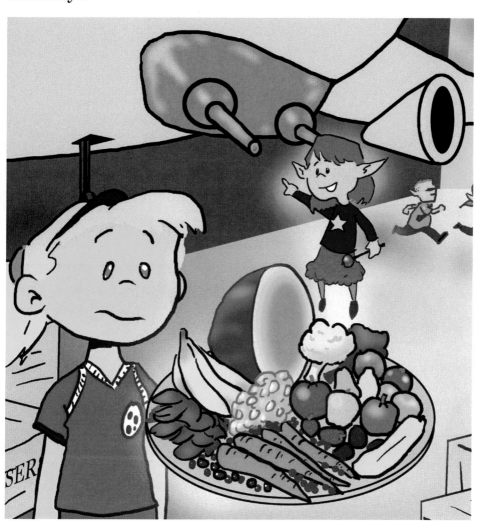

"So eat up, Lucie! The Pilot Elves need lasers!"
Lucie stared at the tray. She made a face at the kale, but grabbed some carrots and broccoli and started eating. It sure didn't taste like candy, but it was crunchy and fresh.

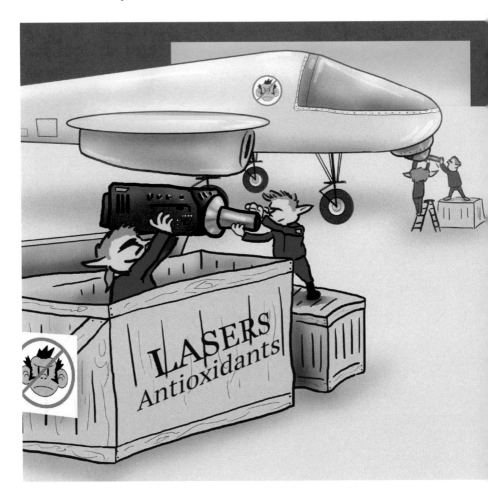

As she chewed, she saw the Rescue Planes pummelling the Mayhem Monkeys with their fabulously-coloured lasers.

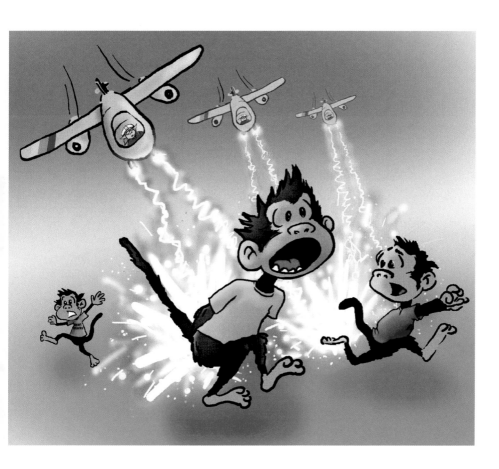

Everyone cheered as the Mayhem Monkeys ran away.

"Hooray!" yelled Lucie. "We did it!"

"No, YOU did it, Lucie" said Stargold. "When you eat fruits and vegetables, your body is better at fighting off bad stuff."

"Ooh! That's why Mommy made me that vegetable omelette."

"Exactly," said Stargold with a big smile. Lucie smiled back.

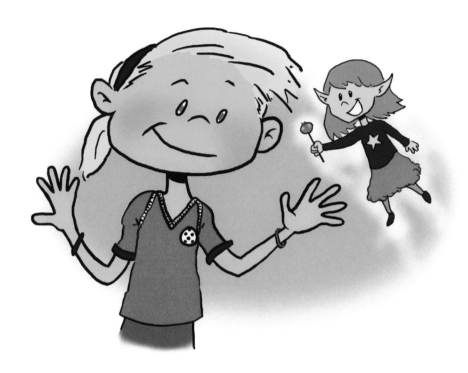

"As you can see," said Stargold, "every last part of your body came from the food you ate. Look at your hands. Look at your feet. Feel your heart beating. These all used to be food!" Lucie stared at her hands in awe.

"Also, listen to your body. It will tell you how much to eat. Treats are fine, as long as you mostly eat the foods that will keep your house strong and healthy."

By then, it was time to go home. Stargold took Lucie's hand and up in the sky they flew.

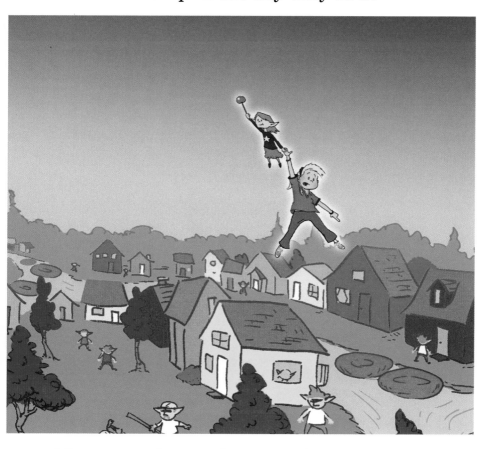

They soared over the giant forest again, flew over the waterfalls, deserts and oceans, to finally arrive back in Lucie's bedroom.

"Thank you so much for showing me Growland," said Lucie. "It was amazing!"

"You are most welcome," said Stargold.

"I will miss you."

"I will miss you too, Lucie," said Stargold.

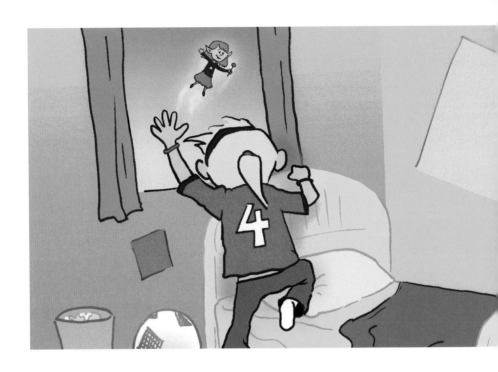

"But we will meet again. In 22 years and 44 days, to be exact, you will need me to talk to your son because he won't eat your veggie pâté."

"No way!" said Lucie. Lucie jumped on her bed and they hugged goodbye. Stargold smiled one last time and left on her rainbow.

Lucie ran back downstairs.

"Mommy, Daddy! I have the most amazing story to tell you! But first, where is that vegetable omellete you made for me!?"

The End

More Stargold Tips:

When picking what to eat, remember that 'fresh is best' and try to choose 'quality over quantity'. But eating is fun and it should remain that way.

Take your time to eat and enjoy food with friends and family. While it is true that parents are not growing anymore, they should still eat healthy because their body keeps making itself anew from the foods they eat every day.

Take good care of your house. Love your house. All houses have one purpose and one purpose only: to host a tiny human being inside, and that's what is really magical. Think of how lucky you are to get a brand new house for free!

You are not your house. You just live in it. All houses are amazing in their own way.

After all, the true meaning of life is not to look at one's own house, but instead to look outside the window. You could be missing a rainbow!

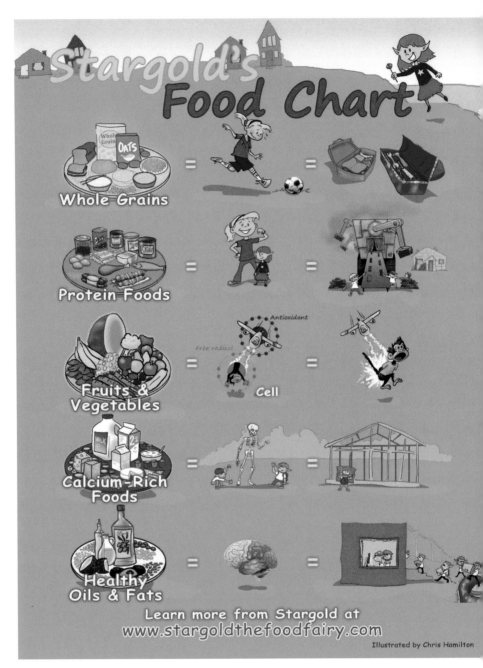

To order copies of "Stargold's Food Chart" in poster format, visit www.stargoldthefoodfairy.com

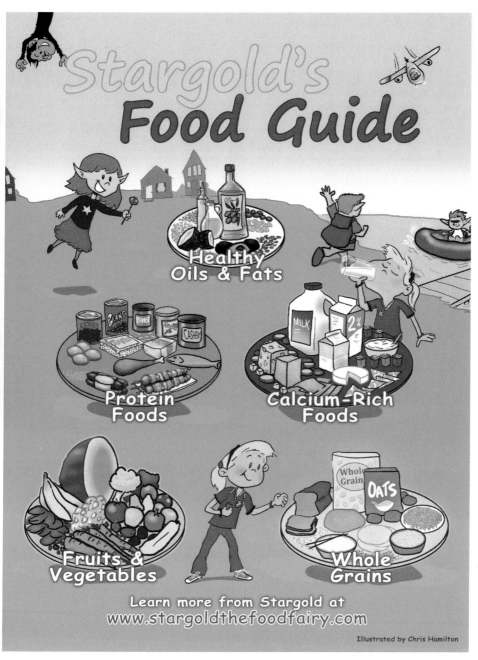

To order copies of "Stargold's Food Guide" in poster format,

visit www.stargoldthefoodfairy.com

Acknowledgements:

- My first big thank you goes to <u>Ellyn Satter,</u> MS RD LCSW BCD, who graciously allowed me to use her "Division of Responsibilities" principles in my book.
- Dr. Linda Starkey, PhD, who did not let me quit when I wanted to.
- Mme. Ginette Caron, MSc, who gave me the possibility to continue when I wanted to.
- Thank you to Katy Quévillon, MA, for turning my "readable" story into an enjoyable one.
- Thank you to Chantel Faucher, PhD, for her editing expertise.
- Thank you to Alicia Coelho for making the book so much better (and shorter!).
- Thank you to <u>Chris Hamilton</u> for making my story look prettier than what I could ever envision myself.
- Thank you to <u>Doug McKinnon</u> for his excellence and patience with me: "One last change, promise!"
- Thank you to my children Justin and Amélie. Justin came up with the name Stargold, and Amélie (who did not want to try my omelette) made me realize that a story needed to be written.
- Thank you most of all to my husband Peter Zakrzewski who encouraged and supported me in following my dreams Thank you for your infinite patience in helping me turn my "unreadable" mess into a "readable story".

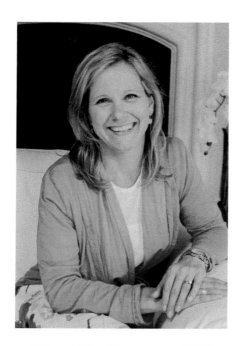

Claudia Lemay, RD
Author

Claudia Lemay resides in Surrey, British Columbia, Canada with her husband, two kids and two pets. She works in a long-term care facility as a clinical dietitian. Claudia also created the program Eat.Go.Grow!, a summer camp for children that encourages healthy nutrition and physical activity.

To learn more about Stargold and healthy nutrition for children, or to find out how to order educational posters or this story in a teacher's presentation version, please visit www.stargoldthefoodfairy.com.

Stargold's Pyramid

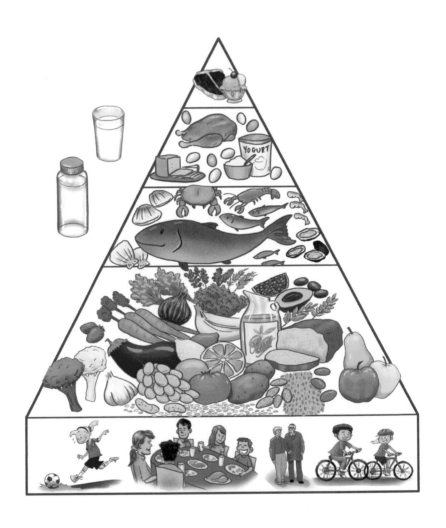

Made in the USA
Monee, IL
10 December 2019

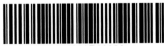